WHAT YOU NEED TO GET STARTED

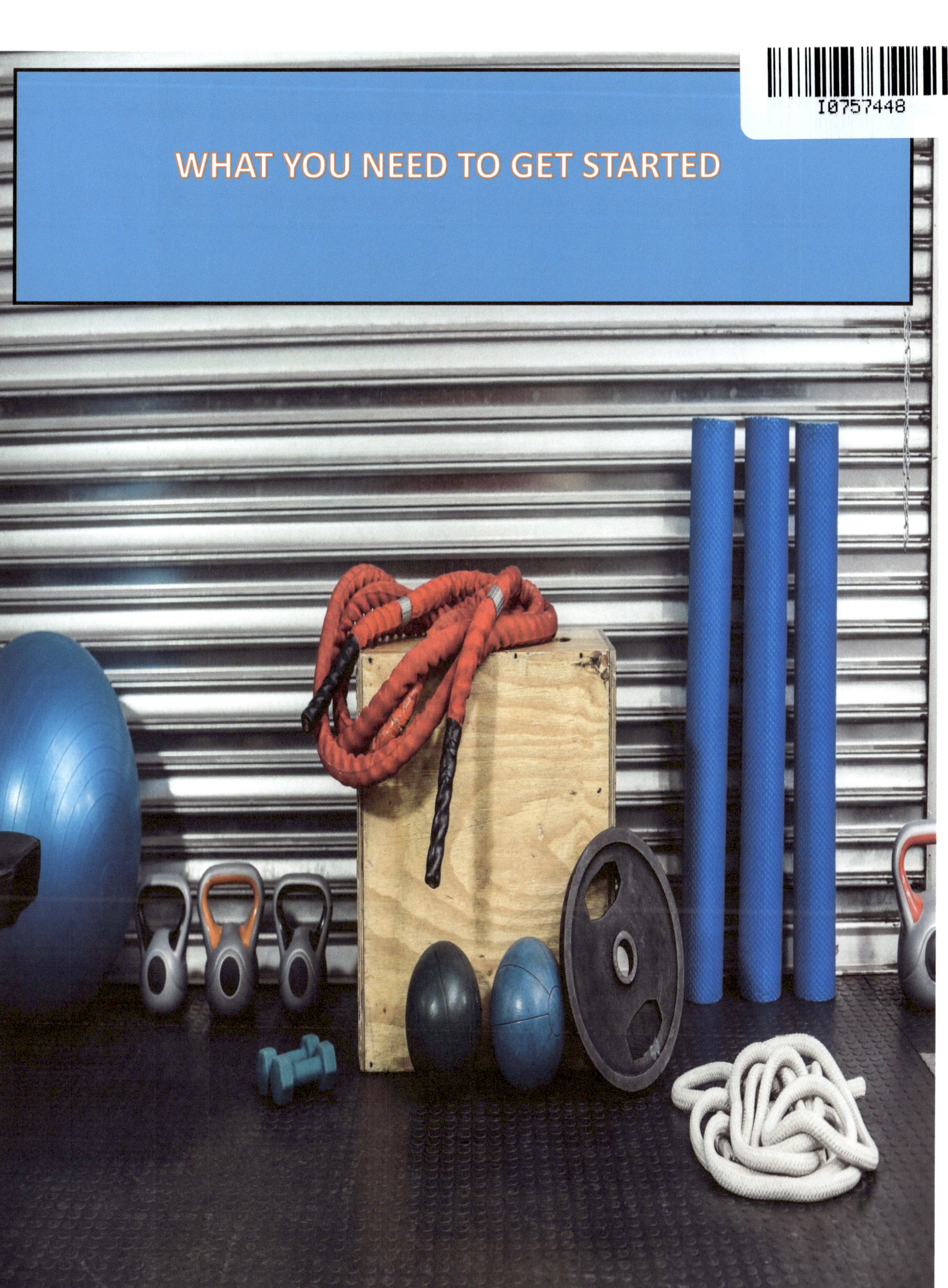

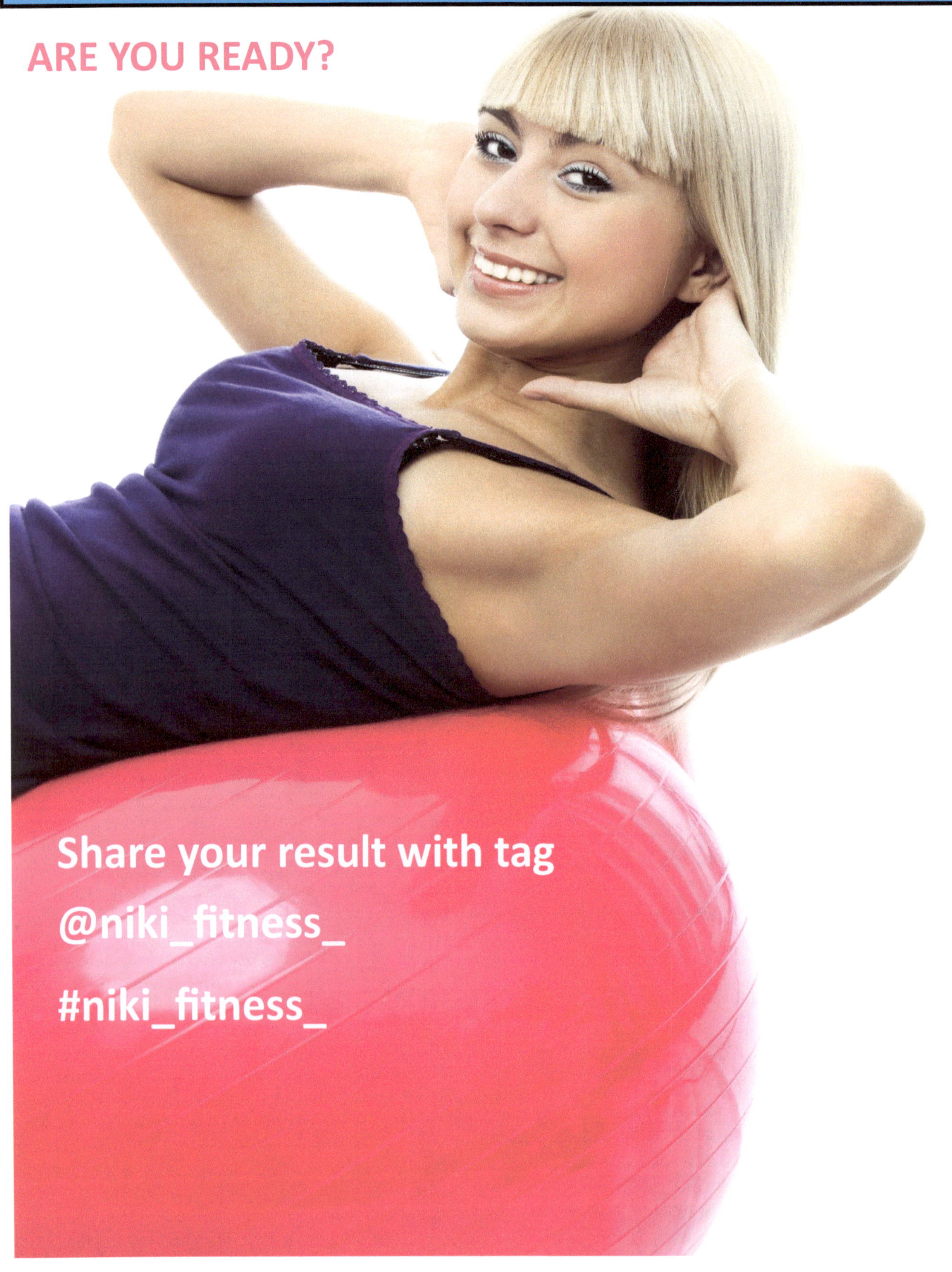

Follow us on Instagram
@niki_fitness_
ARE YOU READY?
Share your result with tag
@niki_fitness_
#niki_fitness_

TABLE OF CONTENT

WEEK 1

MONDAY HIIT

FULL BODY

REST(BETWEEN EACH HIIT CIRCUILT).3 MINTS.BEGAIN HIT CIRCULT AGIAN

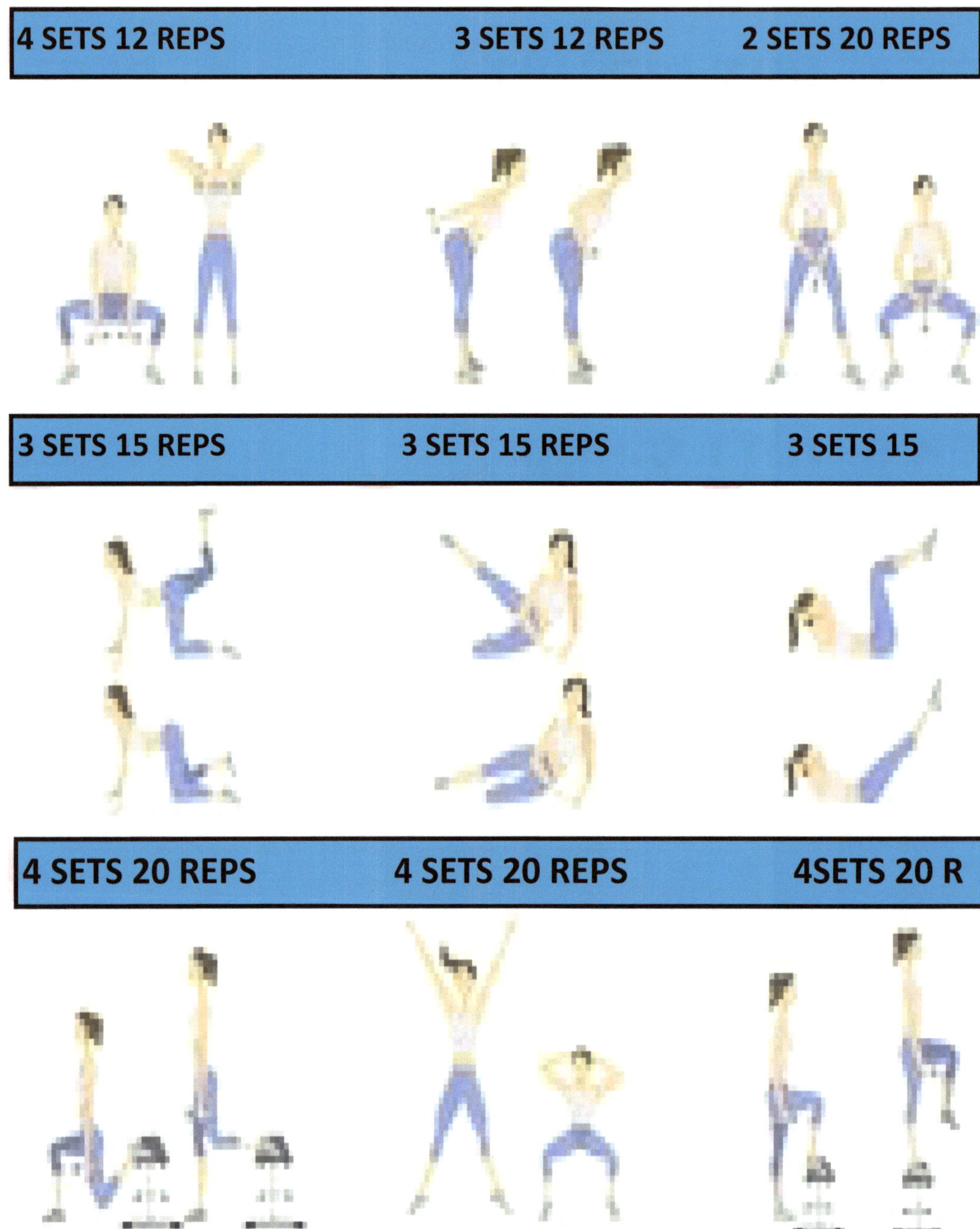

4 SETS 12 REPS
3 SETS 12 REPS
2 SETS 20 REPS
3 SETS 15 REPS
3 SETS 15 REPS
3 SETS 15
4 SETS 20 REPS
4 SETS 20 REPS
4SETS 20 R

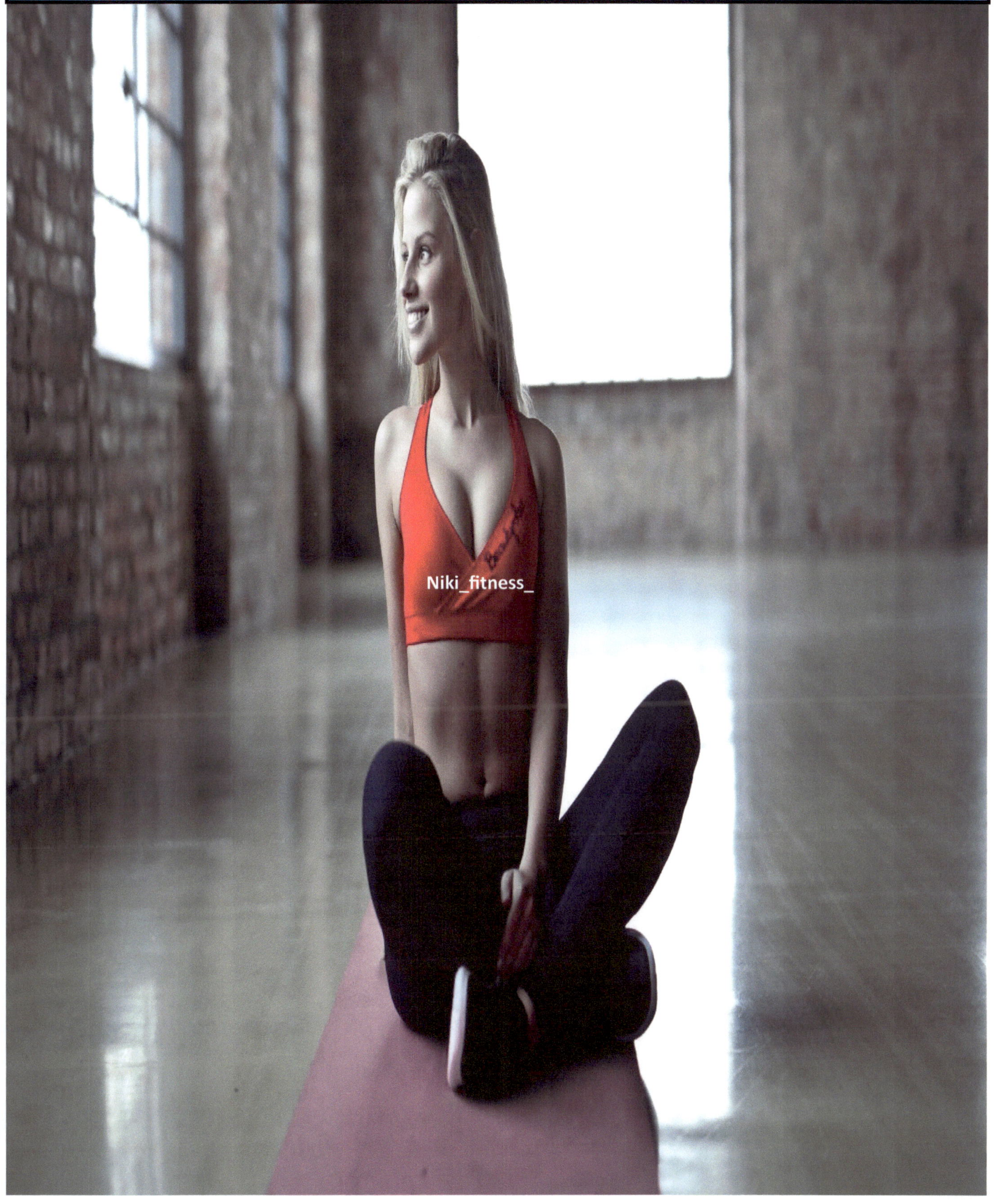
Niki_fitness_

TUESDAY HIIT

FULL BODY

REST(BETWEEN EACH HIIT CIRCUILT).3 MINTS.BEGAIN HIT CIRCULT AGIAN

12 PUSH UP	3SETS 10REPS	2SETS 10 REPS

3 SETS 7REPS	20 SHRUG	20 PUSHUP

3 SETS 12 REPS	5 SETS 10SETS	2SETS 20 REPS

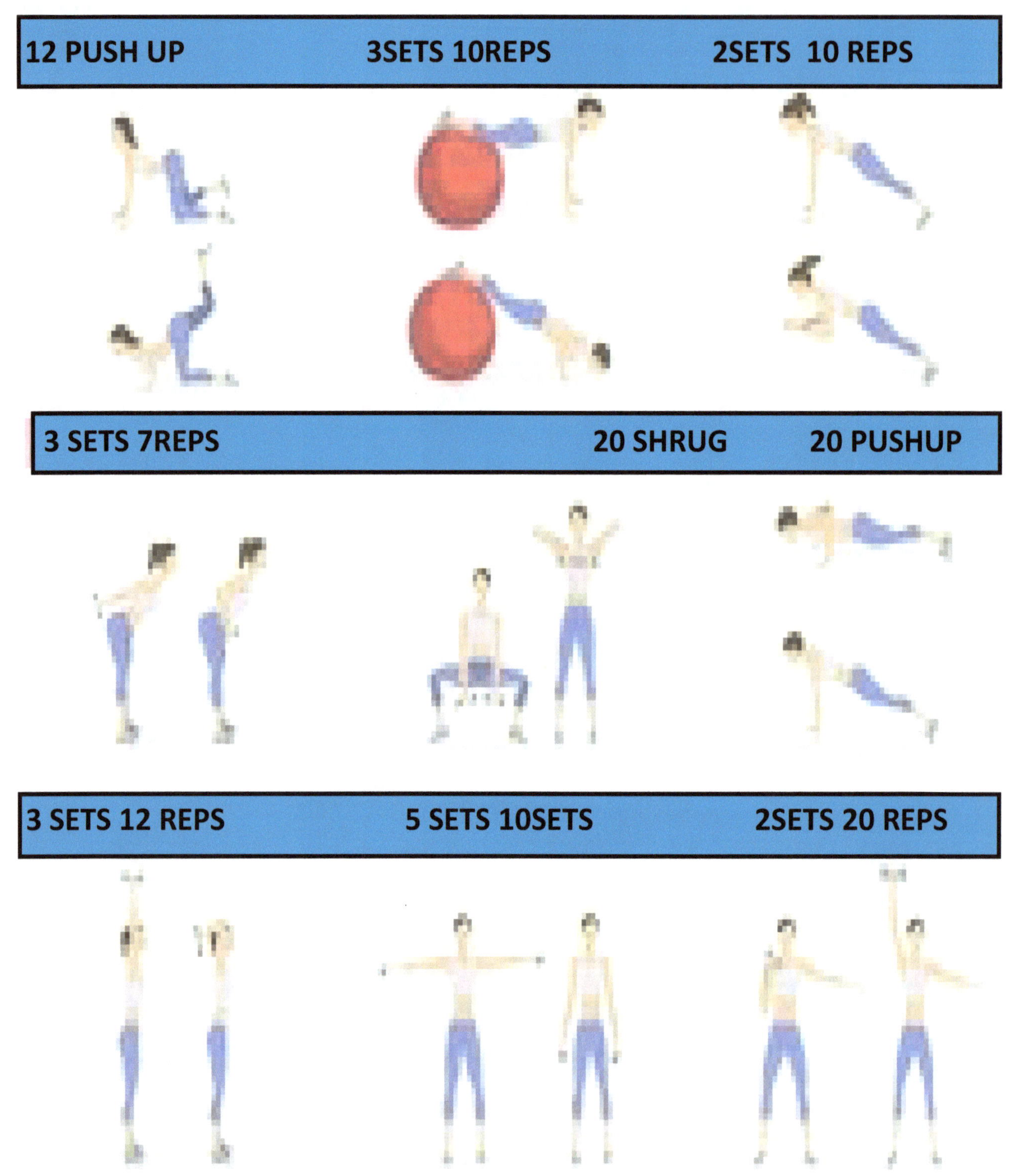

<table><tr><td>WEEK 3</td><td>WEDNDAY HIIT

FULL BODY

REST(BETWEEN EACH HIIT CIRCUILT).3 MINTS.BEGAIN HIT CIRCULT AGIAN</td></tr></table>

3 SETS 15 REPS KICKBACK | **2 SETS 15 REPS** | **4 SET   12**

20 SUMO SQUAT | **4 SETS 12 REPS** | **4 SETS   15 REPS**

20 SUMO SQUAT | **3 SETS 12 REPS** | **4 SETS 20 REPS**

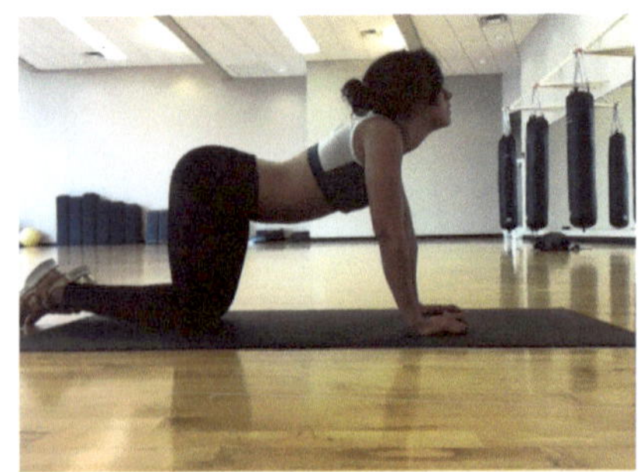

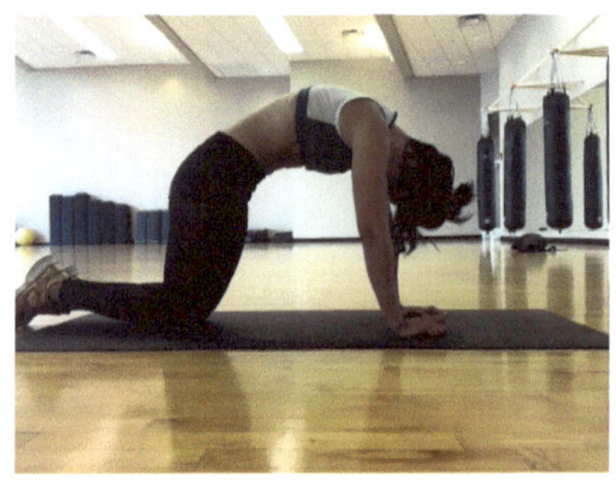

1.CAT-COW

3 SETS OF 6 REPS

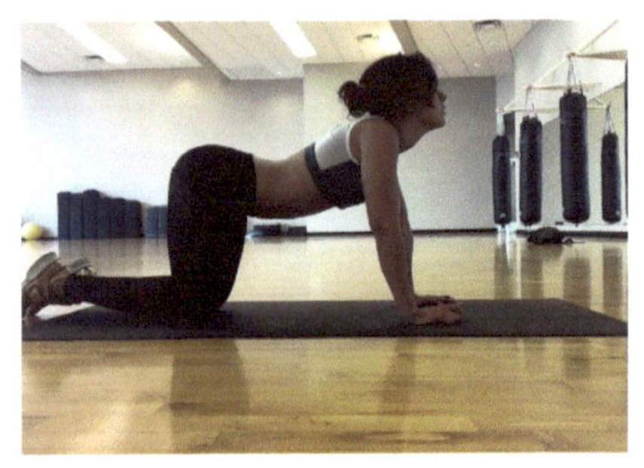

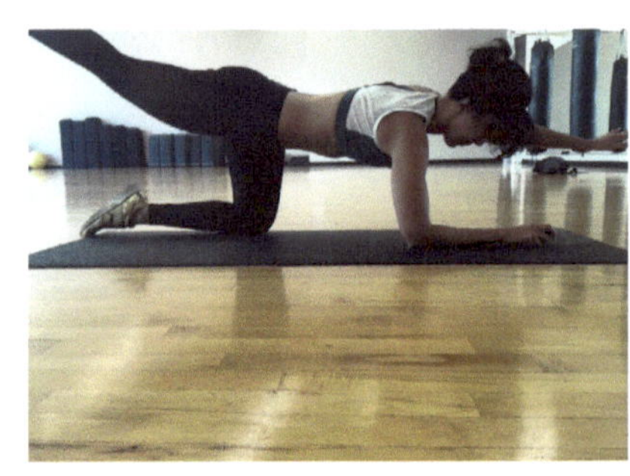

2.OPPOSIT ARM AND LEG BALANCE

4 SETS OF 8 REPS

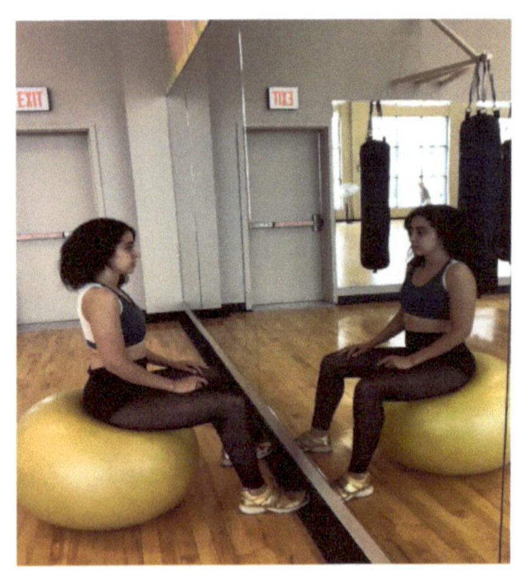

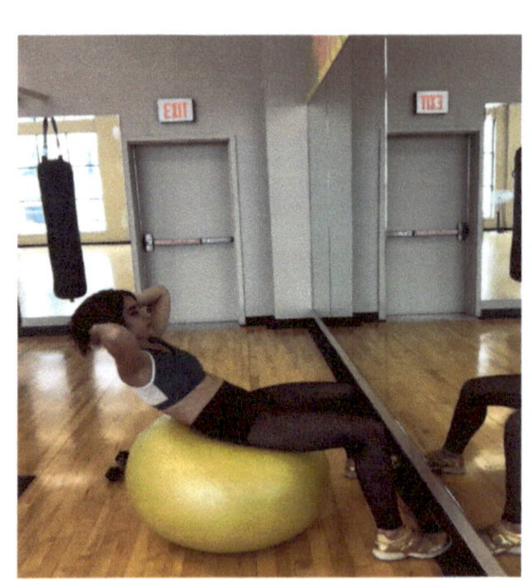

3.AB CRUNCH ON STABLITY BALL   3 SETS OF 6 REPS

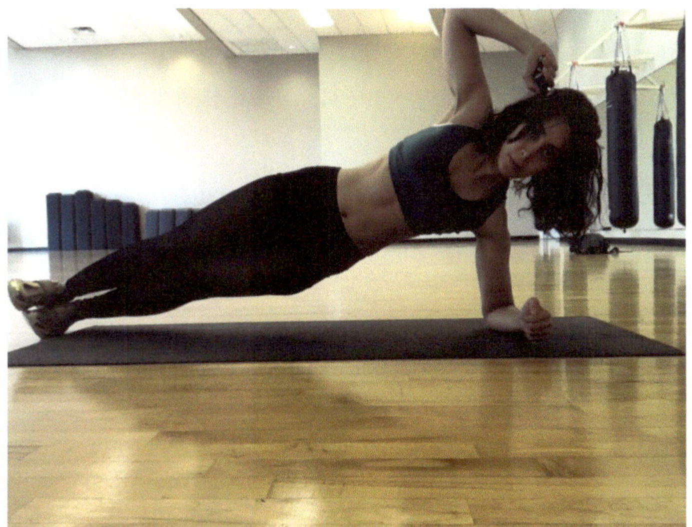

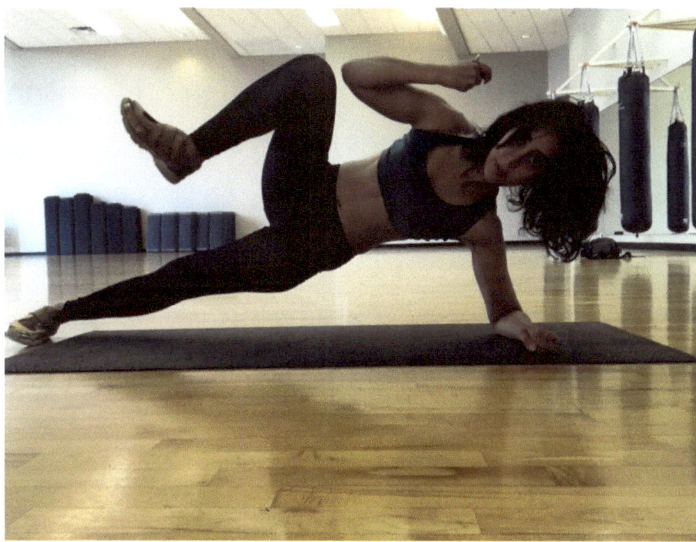

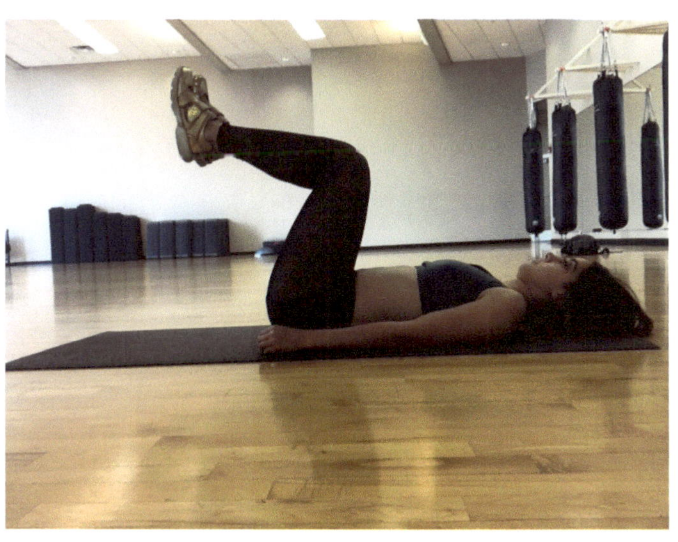

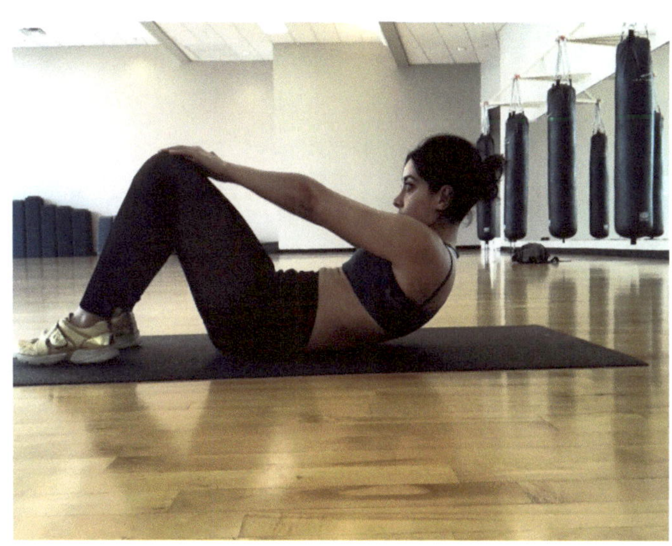

How to Do Cat-Cow Pose

gentle warm-up sequence. When practiced together, the poses help to stretch the body and prepare it for other activity.

Benefits of Cat-Cow

This sequence also helps to develop postural awareness and balance throughout the body. It brings the spine into correct alignment and can help prevent back pain when practiced regularly.

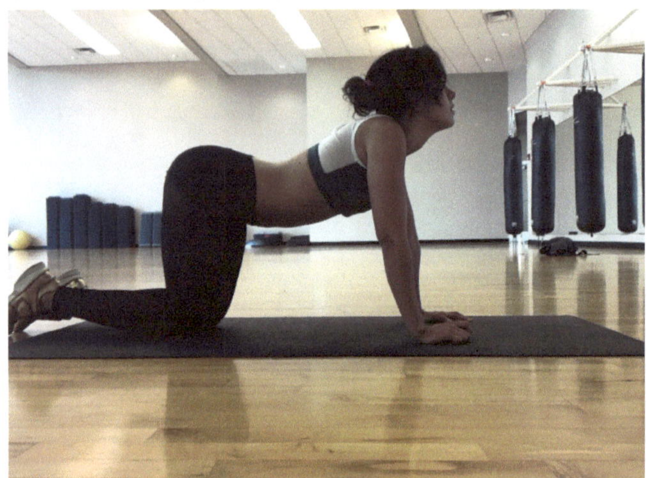 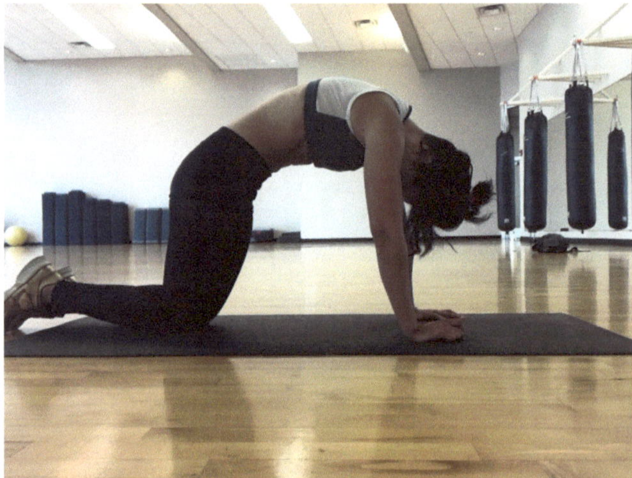

1. Start on your hands and knees with your wrists directly under your shoulders, and your knees directly under your hips. Point your fingertips to the top of your mat. Place your shins and knees hip-width apart. Center your head in a neutral position and soften your gaze downward.

2. Begin by moving into Cow Pose: Inhale as you drop your belly towards the mat. Lift your chin and chest, and gaze up toward the ceiling.

3. Broaden across your shoulder blades and draw your shoulders away from your ears.

4. Next, move into Cat Pose: As you exhale, draw your belly to your spine and round your back toward the ceiling. The pose should look like a cat stretching its back.

5. Release the crown of your head toward the floor, but don't force your chin to your chest.

6. Inhale, coming back into Cow Pose, and then exhale as you return to Cat Pose. Repeat 5-20 times, .

Opposite Arm and Leg Balance

Get down on the floor with your hands completely straight and under your shoulders. Your knees should be bent to 90 degrees, placing them directly beneath your

Tighten your core and extend one arm forward so that your shoulder is next to your ear. At the same time, straighten your opposite leg completely behind you, bringing it to hip height. Return to the starting position and repeat with your opposite arm and leg.

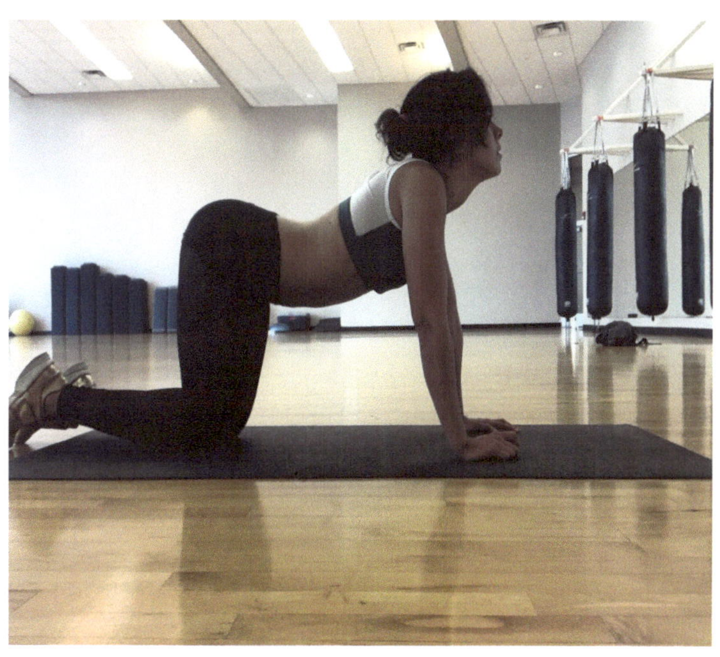

TIPS

Avoid overarching your back at the top of the movement. Focus on maintaining a neutral spine throughout the exercise.
Don't allow your hips to shift side to side during the exercise.
As you extend your leg back make sure you squeeze your glutes for added stability.

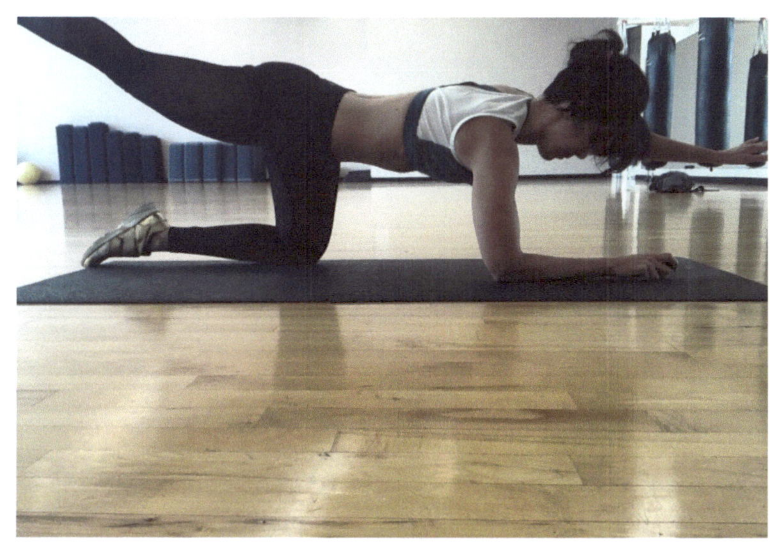

1-Start by lying on your back with your knees bent

2-Put your in front of you and tall

3-Lift your torso up as close to your thighs as possible.

4-Lower your torso down to the floor so you're back in the starting position.

5-Do 3 sets of 10-15 reps

2 BENEFITS OF THE SIT UPS EXERCISE

The sit up has a great range of motion so not only does it work your abdominals it also works your hips too, helping to build a strong core.
It requires no equipment apart from a mat and a small amount of space.

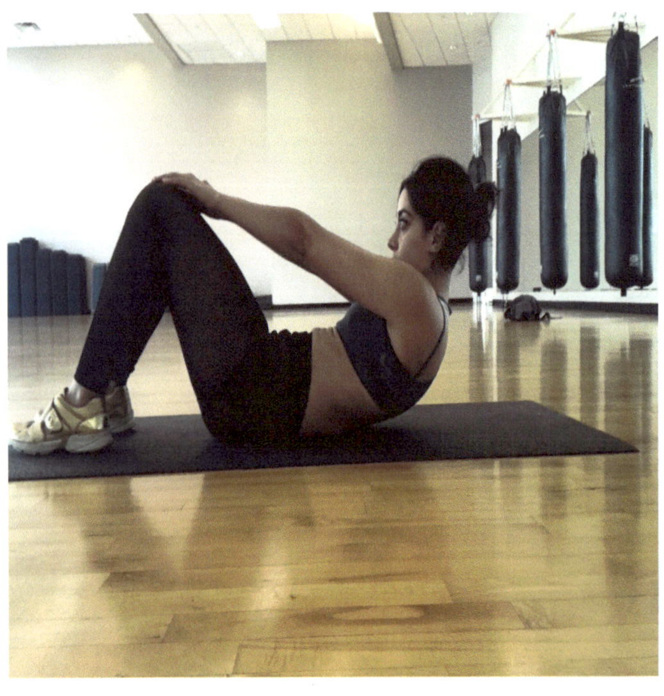 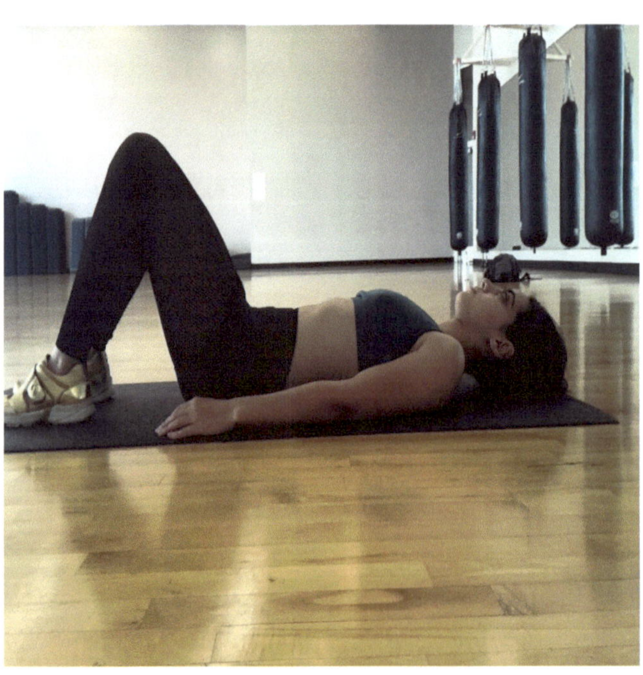

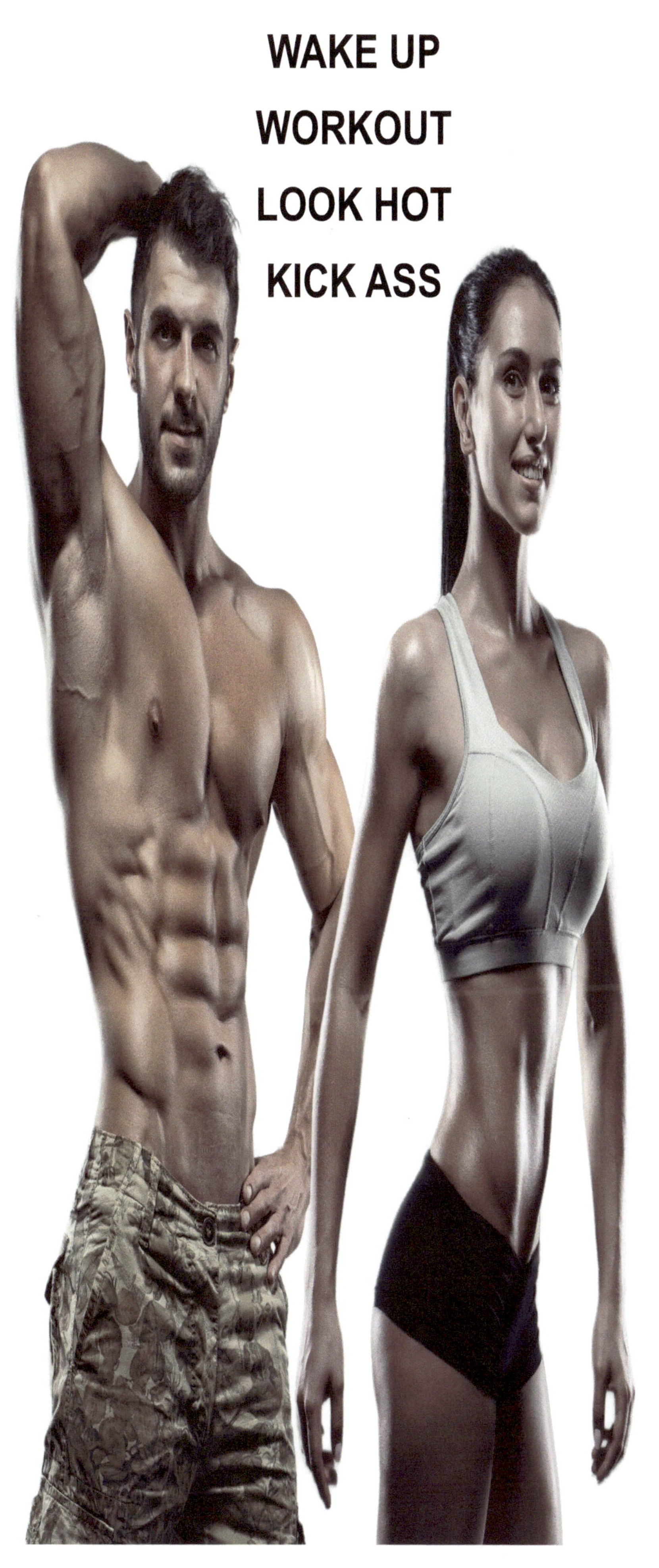

WAKE UP
WORKOUT
LOOK HOT
KICK ASS

Hip Thrust
BENIFIT

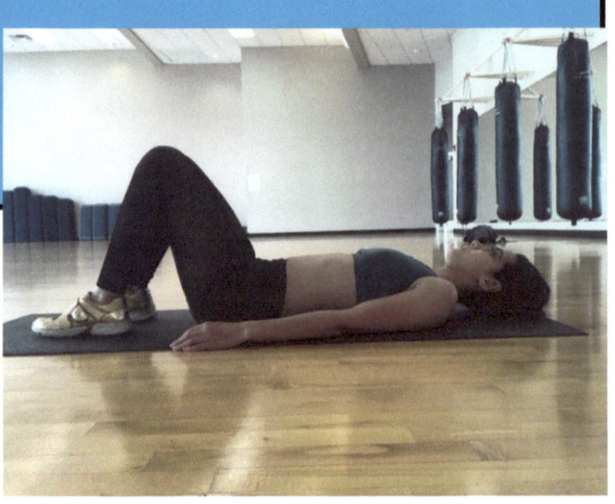

the **Hip Thrust** is a glute exercise designed to improve your strength, speed and power by teaching optimal **hip** extension. ... The glutes are designed to extend the **hip** or pull the leg behind the body. If your glutes are underdeveloped, your speed, power and strength are all compromised.

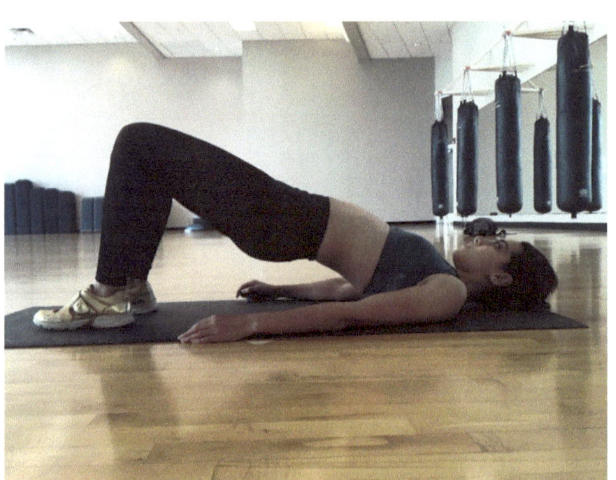

HOW TO DO HIP THRUST

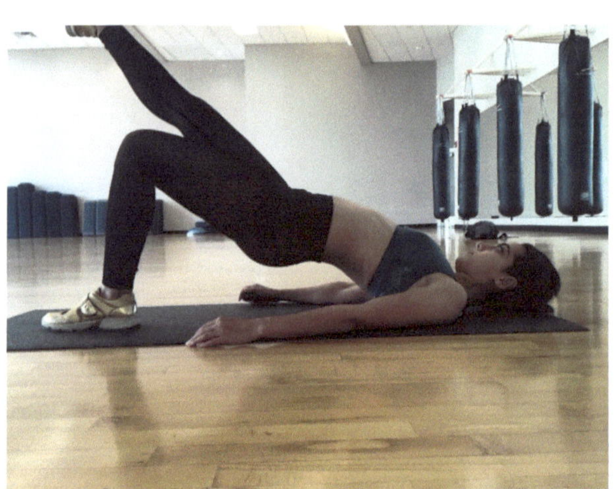

1. Start with your shoulder blades against a bench, and your arms spread across it for stability. ...
2. Take a big breath in, blow your air out fully, and brace your core.
Squeeze your glutes, lift up your hips, and hold a second or two.

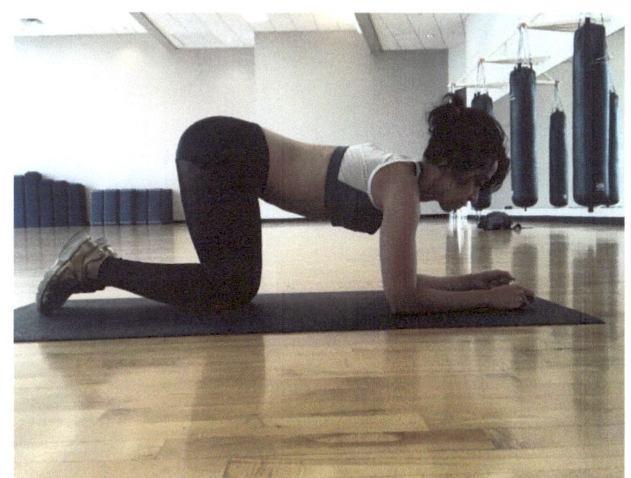 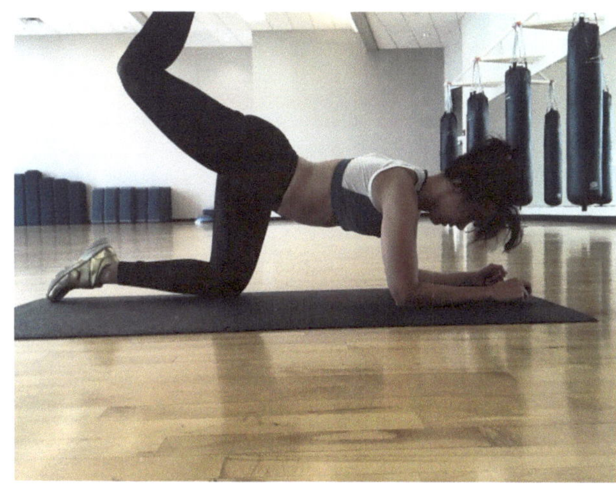

How to Do Glute Kickbacks

1. Kneeling on a mat with forearms propping up your torso. Place a dumbbell behind one knee and keep it bent to hold the dumbbell in place. Tighten abs to engage your abdominals to stabilize yourself during the exercise. Coaching Key: -Your shoulders should be directly above the elbows. (your elbows need to be at 90 degree angle).
2. Lift up the weighted leg up to the point that you form a straight line from your shoulder, butt, and knee. Coaching Key: -Your thigh should be parallel to the floor.
3. Return to the starting position, but don't let your weighted knee touch and rest on the ground. Repeat 10 times. Switch legs and repeat.

Target Muscles:

- Butt
- Hamstrings
- Lower Back
- Core

IT COMES DOWN TO ONE SINGLE THING

HOW BAD DO YOU WANTIT?

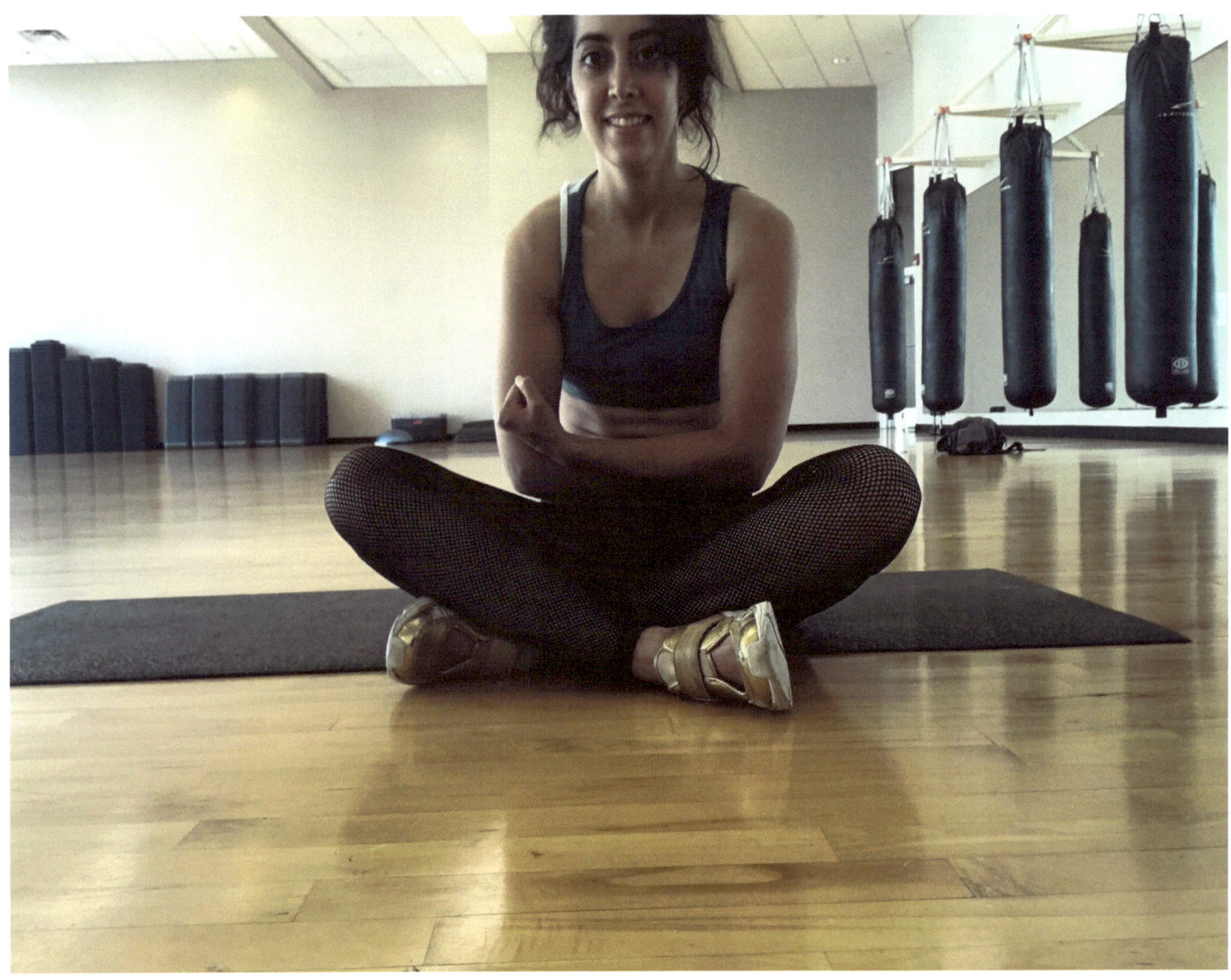

Dumbbell plank row

- Start in a plank position with your legs wider than hip-width distance; the wider stance makes you more stable. Hold onto your dumbbells, keeping your wrist locked to protect the joint.

- With your core tight and your glutes engaged, exhale, stabilizing your torso as you lift your right elbow to row; feel your right scapula sliding toward your spine as you bend your elbow up toward the ceiling.

- Keeping your neck long and energized, return the weight to the ground and re-

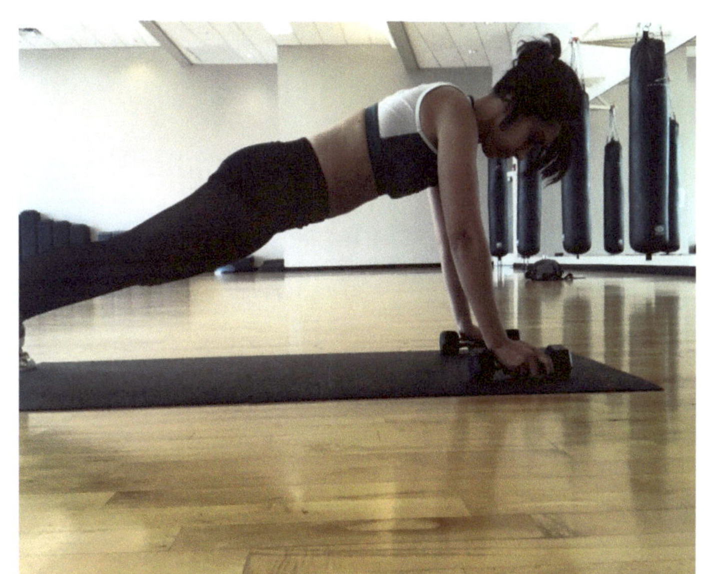

benefit

Fat Attack Exercise for Core and Back: **Plank** Position **Dumbbell Row**.
The **plank** position **dumbbell row** (also known as the renegade **row**), is a challenging exercise that builds rock hard strength in the abdominals (core), upper back, biceps, triceps and shoulders.

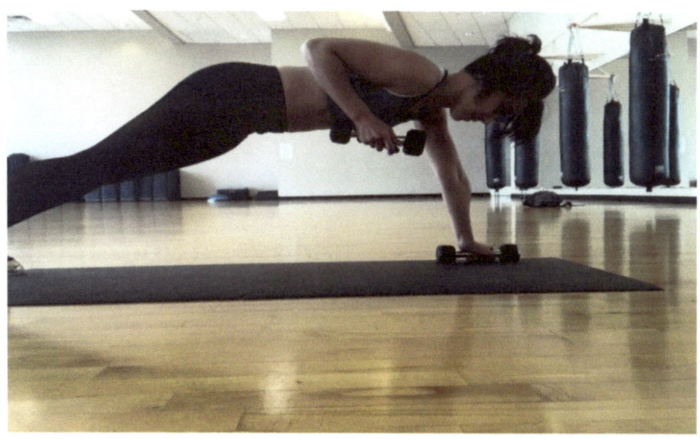

- Begin in Positive Seated Posture; roll out until lower back is resting comfortably on ball.

- Place feet flat on floor, shoulder-width apart.

- Position hands behind head to support its weight, elbows pointing directly out to sides.

- Raise head even with torso and gaze straight up.

- Inhale deeply; on exhale, contract lower abs.

- Hold the flex and inhale; on exhale, slowly curl torso forward, flexing middle and upper abs to raise chest up and toward pelvis. Allow head to follow chest. Do not force or pull head forward. Allow abs to do the work.

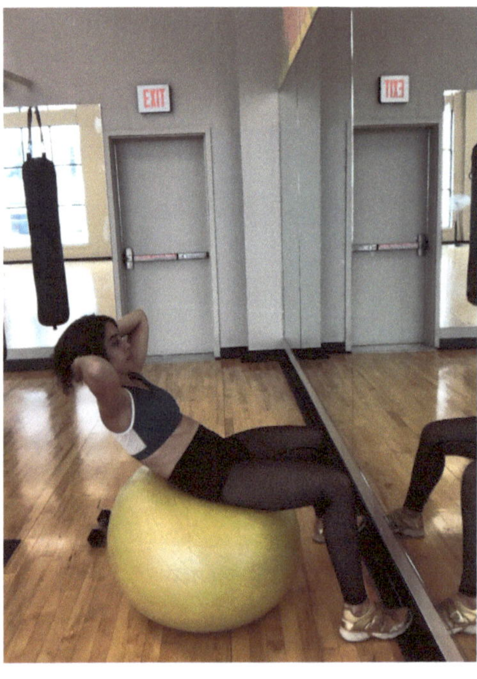
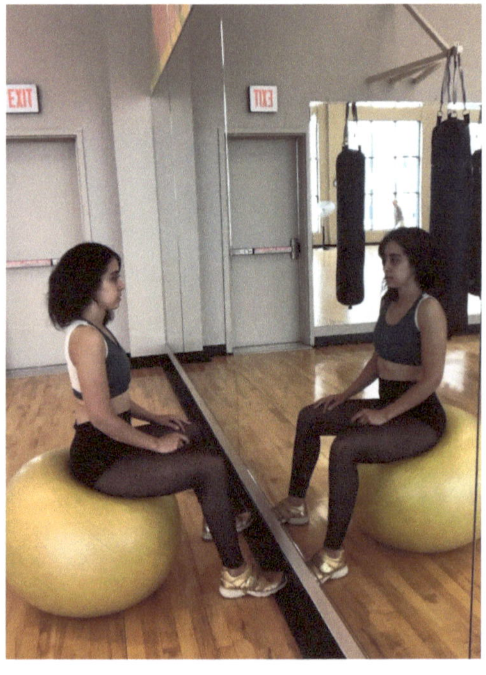

BENIFITS

The **stability ball crunch** is an **abdominal exercise** which predominantly targets the-**abdominal** muscles. It's a progression from doing **crunches** on the floor, on a mat be-cause additional **core strength** and **stability** is required to **balance** on the**ball**

Easy Chicken and Rice Casserole

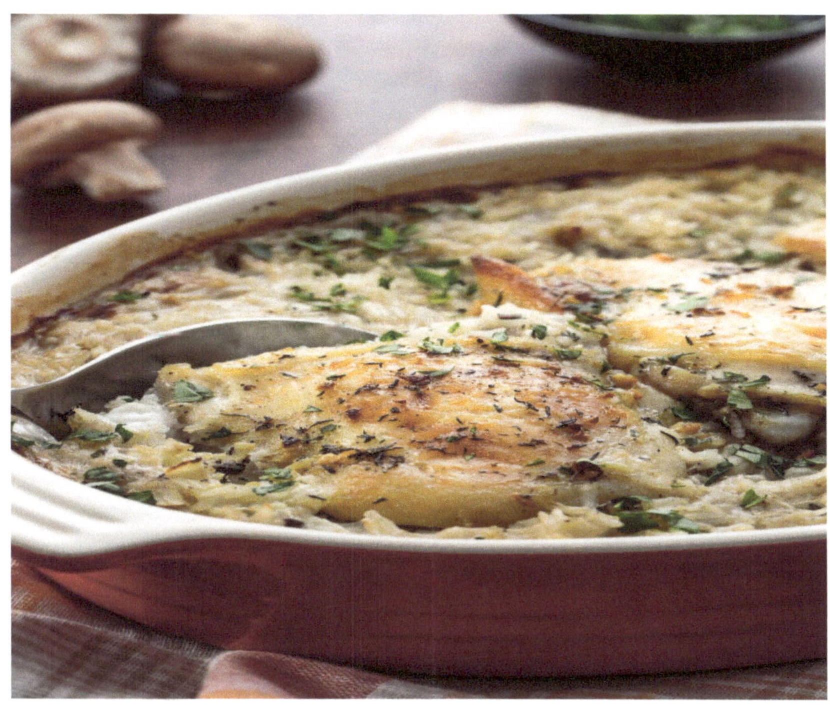

Easy Chicken and Rice Casserole

INGREDIANT

Extra-virgin olive oil, for baking dish

2 c. white rice

1 large onion, chopped

2 c. low-sodium chicken broth

Freshly ground black pepper

3 large bone-in, skin-on chicken thighs

1 clove garlic, finely minced

1 tbsp. Freshly chopped parsley, for garnish

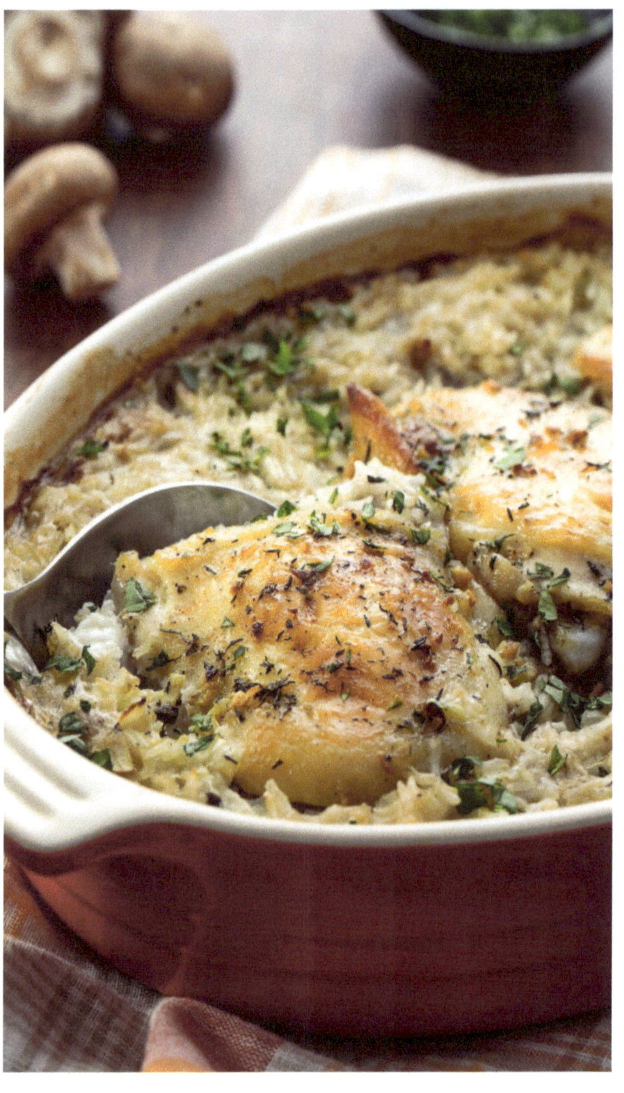

1. Preheat oven to 350° and grease a 9"-x-13" baking dish with oil. Add rice, onion, broth, and soup and stir until combined. Season with salt and pepper.
2. Place chicken thighs in rice mixture and brush with melted butter. Sprinkle with thyme and garlic and season with salt and pepper.
3. Cover dish with foil and bake for 1 hour. Uncover and bake 30 minutes more, until rice is cooked and chicken is golden

Garnish with parsley before serving.

Watermelon slushies

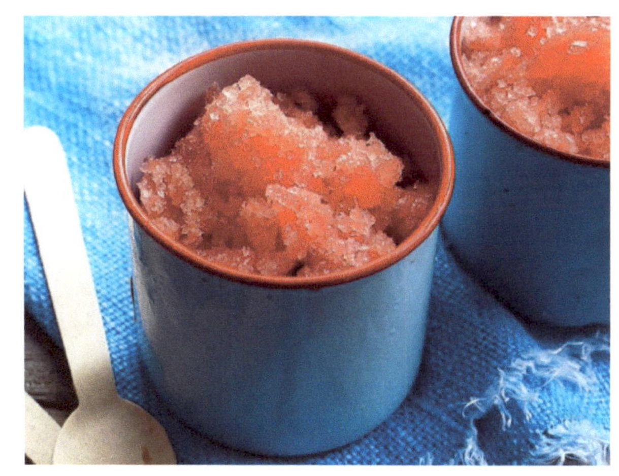

INGREDIENTS

- 10 cups Seedless Watermelon Cubes, frozen for at least 24 hours
- 2-4 tbsp. Maple Syrup*
- Juice of 1 large Lime
- 1/4 cup Fresh Mint or Basil leaves, loosely packed (*Optional, but recommended*)
- 1 1/2 cup Filtered Water (*see notes for a fun substitution!*)

INSTRUCTIONS

1. First, let the Frozen Watermelon chunks sit at room temperature for 5-10 minutes to defrost some. Then, add the Watermelon, 2 tbsp Maple Syrup, Lime Juice, Mint, and Water to a high-speed blender.

2. Pulse the blender until the Watermelon starts to break up some, then blend to form a thick, slushie consistency. Adjust the Maple Syrup to taste, adding more if necessary. If the mixture is too thick for your liking, you can also add in extra water.

Coconut, Cherry and Vanilla

Juicy cherries, creamy coconut milk and a generous amount of vanilla come together to create a delicious frozen dessert that's ideal for scorching days. These are not your regular ice pops, loaded with refined sugar: Small amounts of honey and maple syrup give just the right amount of sweetness and add flavor.

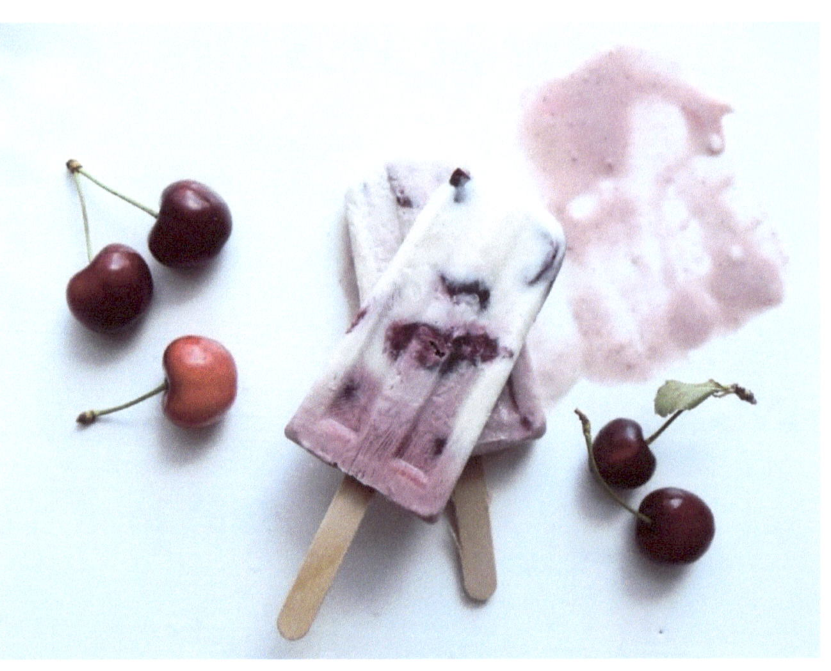

Watermelon Slushies

This sweet treat is a great make-ahead item for summer parties, and it couldn't be easier to prepare — just puree and freeze watermelon.

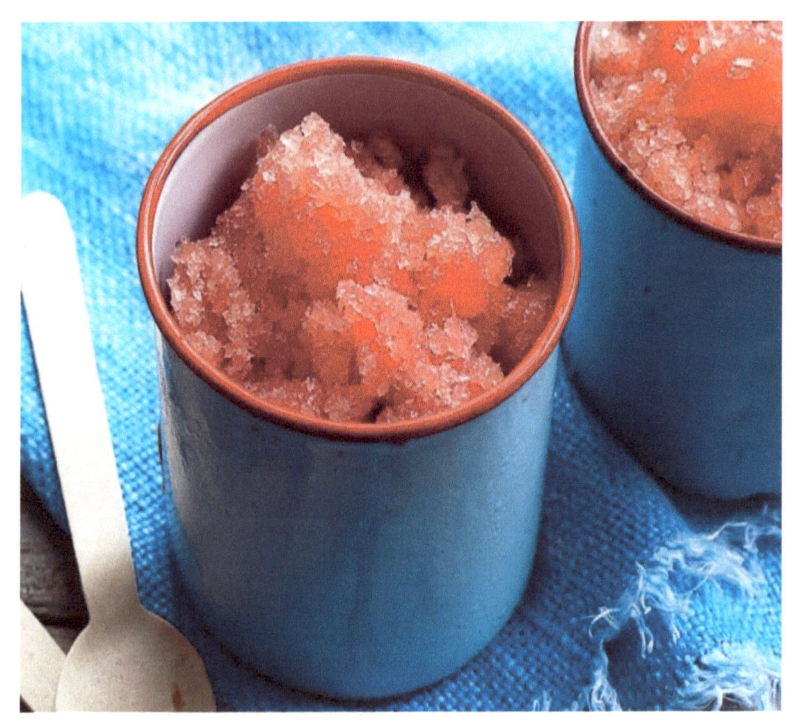

Coconut, Cherry and Vanilla

This sweet treat is a great make-ahead item for summer parties, and it couldn't be easier to prepare — just puree and freeze watermelon.

Ingredients

2 cups fresh sweet cherries, such as Bing, pitted and halved

2 tablespoons pure maple syrup

Pinch cinnamon

3 to 4 drops almond extract

3 to 4 drops almond extract

2 cans full-fat coconut milk

1 vanilla bean, seeds scraped and pod reserved

1 tablespoon pure vanilla extract

3 tablespoons raw honey

1-Bring the cherries, maple syrup, cinnamon and almond extract to a simmer in a small pot over high heat. Cover the pot, reduce the heat to low and simmer until the cherries are juicy and soft, 10 to 15 minutes. Remove the pot from the heat, and set aside.

2-In another small-to-medium pot, bring the coconut milk and vanilla bean seeds and pods to a simmer over high heat, whisking occasionally. Reduce the heat to low, cover the pot and simmer for 5 minutes. Remove from the heat, let cool for 5 minutes, then whisk in the honey and vanilla extract. Remove and reserve the vanilla bean pod. Pour the mixture into a pitcher or measuring jug and set aside.

3-Place a strainer over the blender jar. Add the cooked cherries, and press out the juice. Add 1/3 of the cherry pulp and 1 cup of the coconut milk mixture, and blend until smooth. You should have about 2 cups of liquid. Refrigerate. Divide the remaining coconut milk mixture among ice pop molds, and place them in the freezer until semifrozen, about 1 hour. Remove them from the freezer, and divide the remaining cherry pulp among the molds. Top with the blended cherry-coconut mixture, place the lids on top, add sticks and freeze until solid, at least 8 hours.

4-To remove the ice pops, dip the molds in warm water for a few seconds, then carefully pull on the sticks to release.

Thank you